Title

The Best Drug That's Not Sold in the Pharmacy

Subtitle

Unlocking the Healing Power of Joy for Lifelong Wellness and Fulfillment

Copyright

considered as professional advice
The author and publisher disclaim
any liability arising directly
or indirectly from the use or
application of any information
contained in this book.

Introduction

 In a world where the pursuit of health and wellness often leads us down the aisles of pharmacies and into the realm of prescription medications, there exists a potent remedy that cannot be found on any shelf or prescribed by any doctor. It is a remedy that transcends the confines of traditional medicine, offering healing and vitality to those who embrace its transformative power. This remedy is joy.

Welcome to "The Joy Prescription: Unlocking the Healing Power Within" by Abraham Hunter. In this groundbreaking book, we embark on a journey to discover the profound impact that joy can have on our physical, emotional, and spiritual well-being. Through a blend of scientific research, personal anecdotes, and practical insights, Hunter invites us to explore the remarkable potential of joy as the ultimate prescription for health and happiness.

As the title suggests, joy is not a commodity that can be purchased in a pharmacy. It is not a pill to be swallowed or a potion to be applied. Instead, joy is an inner state of being—a radiant energy that emanates from within and infuses every aspect of our lives with meaning and vitality. Drawing upon centuries-old wisdom traditions, modern psychology, and the latest advances in neuroscience, Hunter reveals the profound ways in which joy can promote healing, resilience, and longevity.

Throughout the pages of this book, we will delve into the science behind joy, exploring how positive emotions impact our immune system, cardiovascular health, and overall longevity. We will uncover the ways in which joy cultivates a sense of connection and belonging, strengthening our relationships and fostering a deeper sense of fulfillment. And we will discover practical strategies for cultivating joy in our daily lives, empowering us to embrace each moment with gratitude, wonder, and resilience.

But "The Joy Prescription" is more than just a manual for achieving happiness; it is a call to reclaim our innate capacity for joy and rediscover the healing power that lies within each of us. As we journey together through these pages, may we awaken to the transformative potential of joy and embrace it as the ultimate prescription for living a life of purpose, vitality, and fulfillment.

Join me on this extraordinary exploration into the heart of joy, where we will uncover the secrets of true healing and unlock the boundless potential that awaits within.

Table Of Contents

"Chapter" (1)

Physical Health

This are step-by-step explanation of how joy can improve physical health:

1. **Positive Emotions and Stress Reduction:**
   - Experiencing joy and other positive emotions can help to reduce stress levels in the body. When you feel joyful, your body releases neurotransmitters such as dopamine and endorphins, which promote feelings of happiness and relaxation.

- Lower stress levels have a positive impact on physical health by reducing the production of stress hormones like cortisol, which, when elevated over time, can contribute to various health problems such as high blood pressure, heart disease, and impaired immune function.

2. **Boosts Immune Function:**
   - Joyful emotions have been associated with a strengthened immune system. Studies have shown that people who experience positive emotions, such as happiness and contentment, tend to have stronger immune responses and are less susceptible

to illnesses like the common cold and flu.

   - Positive emotions may enhance immune function by reducing inflammation in the body and promoting the production of antibodies and immune cells that help to fight off infections and diseases.

3. **Promotes Heart Health:**
   . Research suggests ... have been linked to improved cardiovascular health. technicaly the felling of happiness is caused by 4 chemicals this chemicals are endorphin, dopamine, serotonin and axytocin When you experience joy, your body releases 4

chemicals that help to relax blood vessels, lower blood pressure, and improve circulation.

   - Chronic stress and negative emotions, on the other hand, can contribute to the development of heart disease by increasing blood pressure, constricting blood vessels, and promoting inflammation in the arteries. By contrast, experiencing joy can help to counteract these negative effects and protect heart health.

4. **Enhances Pain Tolerance:**
   - Joyful emotions have been shown to increase pain tolerance and reduce the perception of pain. When you experience joy, your

body releases endorphins, which are natural pain relievers that can help to alleviate discomfort and reduce pain sensitivity.

   - Additionally, joyful emotions can distract from pain and provide a sense of relief and well-being, making it easier to cope with chronic pain conditions and other sources of physical discomfort.

5. **Encourages Healthy Lifestyle Behaviors:**
   - Experiencing joy is often associated with engaging in healthy lifestyle behaviors such as regular exercise, nutritious eating, and adequate sleep. When you feel joyful and optimistic, you're more

likely to take care of your physical health and prioritize self-care.

- Positive emotions can motivate you to adopt healthier habits and stick to them over time, leading to better overall health outcomes and a reduced risk of chronic diseases.

6. **Improves Sleep Quality:**
- Joyful emotions can contribute to better sleep quality and duration. When you feel happy and content, your body and mind are more relaxed, making it easier to fall asleep and stay asleep throughout the night.

- Conversely, feelings of stress, anxiety, or sadness can interfere with sleep by causing racing thoughts, muscle tension, and disruptions to the sleep cycle. By cultivating joy and positive emotions, you can promote healthier sleep patterns and improve overall well-being.

7. **Longevity and Life Satisfaction:**

   - Research suggests that experiencing joy and happiness may contribute to a longer life and greater overall life satisfaction. People who report higher levels of happiness tend to live longer, healthier lives compared to those who are less happy.

   - Joyful individuals are more likely to engage in behaviors that promote longevity, such as maintaining strong social connections, engaging in regular physical activity, and adopting healthy eating habits. Additionally, experiencing joy can enhance resilience and coping skills, helping individuals to better navigate life's challenges and maintain a positive outlook as they age.

8. **Reduction in Inflammation:**
- Joyful emotions have been associated with reduced levels of inflammation in the body Studies have found that experiencing positive emotions, such as joy and happiness, can help to lower inflammation in the body, leading to

better overall health and a reduced risk of inflammatory-related diseases.

9. **Enhanced Cognitive Function:**
   - Joyful emotions can positively impact cognitive function and brain health. Research suggests that experiencing positive emotions may improve memory, concentration, and problem-solving abilities.
   - Additionally, joyful individuals may have a lower risk of cognitive decline and dementia in older age, as positive emotions have been associated with better brain health

and resilience against age-related cognitive decline.

10. **Improved Resilience and Coping Skills:**
   - Experiencing joy and happiness can enhance resilience and coping skills, helping individuals to better manage stress and adversity. Joyful individuals tend to approach challenges with optimism and a sense of humor, which can help to buffer against the negative effects of stress on physical health.
   - Cultivating joy and positive emotions can build emotional resilience over time, enabling individuals to bounce back more

quickly from setbacks and maintain a sense of well-being even in the face of adversity.

11. **Social Support and Connection:**
   - Joyful emotions are often experienced in the context of social interactions and connections with others. Strong social support networks have been linked to better physical health outcomes, including lower rates of chronic disease and longer life expectancy.
   - Joyful individuals tend to have stronger social connections and more fulfilling relationships, which can provide emotional support, practical assistance, and a sense

of belonging—all of which contribute to better physical health and well-being.

12. **Mind-Body Connection:**
   - The mind-body connection plays a crucial role in the link between joy and physical health. Positive emotions can influence physiological processes in the body, including hormone regulation, immune function, and cardiovascular health.
   - Conversely, negative emotions such as stress, anxiety, and depression can have detrimental effects on physical health by disrupting these same physiological processes. By

cultivating joy and positive emotions, individuals can promote harmony between the mind and body, leading to better overall health outcomes.

Incorporating these additional aspects into our understanding of the link between joy and physical health further highlights the profound impact that positive emotions can have on our well-being. By prioritizing joy and cultivating a positive outlook, we can enhance not only our physical health but also our overall quality of life.

In summary, joy is closely linked with physical health in numerous ways, including stress reduction, immune enhancement, heart health promotion, pain tolerance improvement, encouragement of healthy lifestyle behaviors, improvement of sleep quality, and promotion of longevity and life satisfaction. Cultivating joy and positive emotions can have profound effects on physical well-being, contributing to a healthier, happier life overall.

"Chapter" (2)

"Joy And Mental Well Being"

Here's are step-by-step exploration of the connection between joy and mental well-being:

1. **Understanding Joy:**

   - Joy is a positive emotion characterized by feelings of happiness, contentment, and inner peace. It is often experienced in response to pleasurable or fulfilling experiences, accomplishments, or moments of gratitude.

2. **Positive Emotions and Mental Health:**

   - Positive emotions, including joy, play a crucial role in promoting mental well-being. They serve as buffers against stress, anxiety, and depression, helping to build resilience and coping skills.

   - Experiencing joy can enhance mood, increase overall life

satisfaction, and contribute to a greater sense of emotional balance and stability.

3. **Neurobiological Basis:**
   - Joyful experiences trigger the release of neurotransmitters such as dopamine, serotonin, and endorphins in the brain. These chemicals are associated with feelings of pleasure, reward, and well-being.
   - Dopamine, in particular, plays a central role in the brain's reward system, reinforcing behaviors associated with pleasure and motivation. Serotonin contributes to feelings of happiness and contentment, while endorphins act

as natural painkillers and mood boosters.

4. **Stress Reduction:**

   - Experiencing joy can help to reduce stress levels by activating the body's relaxation response. When you feel joyful, your body releases hormones that counteract the effects of stress hormones like cortisol, promoting feelings of relaxation and calmness.

   - Regular experiences of joy and positive emotions can help to lower overall stress levels and mitigate the harmful effects of chronic stress on mental health.

5. **Enhanced Resilience:**

- Joyful individuals tend to have greater resilience and coping skills, allowing them to bounce back more quickly from setbacks and adversity. Positive emotions help to broaden cognitive and behavioral repertoires, enabling individuals to consider a wider range of solutions to problems.

- Joy fosters a sense of optimism and hope, even in challenging circumstances, which can help individuals maintain a positive outlook and persevere through difficult times.

6. **Improved Relationships:**
- Experiencing joy can enhance interpersonal relationships and

social connections. Joyful individuals are more likely to engage in positive social interactions, express empathy and kindness towards others, and build strong, supportive relationships.

   - Positive emotions create a ripple effect, leading to greater harmony and cooperation in relationships and fostering a sense of connection and belonging within social networks.

7. **Sense of Purpose and Meaning:**
   - Joy is often associated with feelings of purpose and meaning in life. Experiencing joy can help individuals to identify and pursue

activities, goals, and relationships that align with their values and passions.

   - By cultivating joy and positive emotions, individuals can find greater satisfaction and fulfillment in their daily lives, leading to a deeper sense of purpose and a greater overall sense of well-being.

8. **Promotes Psychological Health:**
   - Experiencing joy is closely linked to psychological health and resilience. Joyful individuals tend to have lower rates of anxiety, depression, and other mental health disorders.

- Positive emotions contribute to greater emotional stability, self-esteem, and self-efficacy, leading to better overall mental health outcomes and a greater capacity to cope with life's challenges.

9. **Mindfulness and Presence:**
   - Joy is often experienced in moments of mindfulness and presence, when individuals are fully engaged in the present moment and appreciative of the beauty and wonder of life.
   - Practicing mindfulness and cultivating a sense of gratitude can help individuals to experience joy more frequently and deeply,

leading to greater mental well-being and life satisfaction.

10. **Long-Term Benefits:**
   - Cultivating joy and positive emotions has long-term benefits for mental health and well-being. Research suggests that individuals who experience higher levels of joy and happiness tend to live longer, healthier lives and have greater overall life satisfaction.
   - By prioritizing joy and incorporating practices that promote positive emotions into daily life, individuals can lay the foundation for lasting mental well-being and resilience.

11. **Enhanced Cognitive Function:**

   - Experiencing joy and positive emotions has been linked to improved cognitive function and mental clarity. When individuals feel joyful, their cognitive processes become more flexible, creative, and efficient.

   - Positive emotions can enhance attention, memory, and problem-solving abilities, leading to better cognitive performance and academic or professional success.

12. **Reduction in Negative Emotions:**

   - Joy serves as a counterbalance to negative

emotions such as sadness, anger, and anxiety. When individuals experience joy, it can help to alleviate and regulate negative emotions, leading to greater emotional balance and stability.

   - Cultivating joy can help individuals develop healthier emotional responses to stressful or challenging situations, allowing them to approach difficulties with optimism and resilience.

13. **Improvement in Mental Health Outcomes:**
   - Research suggests that experiencing joy and positive emotions can have a protective effect against mental health

disorders such as depression and anxiety. Joyful individuals tend to have lower rates of psychological distress and are more resilient in the face of adversity.

- Interventions aimed at promoting joy and positive emotions, such as gratitude exercises, mindfulness practices, and acts of kindness, have been shown to improve mental health outcomes and reduce symptoms of depression and anxiety.

14. **Boost in Self-Esteem and Confidence:**
- Experiencing joy and positive emotions can boost self-esteem and confidence. Joyful individuals

tend to have a more positive self-image and greater self-assurance, leading to improved overall well-being and a greater sense of empowerment.

   - Positive emotions foster a sense of optimism and belief in one's abilities, allowing individuals to approach challenges with confidence and resilience.

15. **Fostering Emotional Intelligence:**

   - Joy can contribute to the development of emotional intelligence, which involves the ability to recognize, understand, and manage one's own emotions as well as those of others. Joyful individuals tend to have greater emotional awareness and empathy, leading to more fulfilling interpersonal relationships and improved communication skills.

   - By cultivating joy and positive emotions, individuals can enhance their emotional intelligence and navigate social interactions with greater ease and effectiveness.

16. **Contribution to Overall Well-Being:**

   - Joy is an essential component of overall well-being, encompassing physical, mental, and emotional aspects of health. When individuals experience joy regularly, it contributes to a sense of holistic well-being and fulfillment.

   - Prioritizing joy and incorporating practices that promote positive emotions into daily life can lead to greater overall well-being, resilience, and life satisfaction.

Incorporating these additional aspects into our understanding of the connection between joy and mental well-being highlights the multifaceted nature of joy and its profound impact on psychological health. By prioritizing joy and cultivating positive emotions, individuals can foster greater mental well-being, resilience, and happiness in their lives.

In summary, joy is closely intertwined with mental well-being, serving as a powerful force for promoting emotional balance, resilience, and life satisfaction. By nurturing joy and positive emotions, individuals can enhance their mental health and cultivate a greater sense of fulfillment and meaning in life.

'Chapter (3)"

The Connection Joy And Relationship

Certainly! Here's a step-by-step exploration of the connection between joy and enhancing relationships:

1. **Understanding Joy in Relationships:**
   - Joy is a positive emotion characterized by feelings of happiness, delight, and fulfillment. In the context of relationships, joy contributes to a sense of connection, intimacy, and mutual happiness between individuals.

2. **Shared Experiences of Joy:**
   - Shared experiences of joy create bonds and strengthen connections between individuals. When people share moments of joy together, whether through laughter,

celebration, or shared achievements, it fosters a sense of closeness and unity in relationships.

3. **Positive Communication:**
   - Joyful individuals are more likely to engage in positive communication with their partners, friends, family members, and colleagues. They express appreciation, gratitude, and affection, leading to greater emotional intimacy and satisfaction in relationships.
   - Positive communication creates a supportive and nurturing environment where individuals feel

valued, understood, and respected by their loved ones.

4. **Emotional Support and Empathy:**
   - Experiencing joy enhances individuals' capacity for empathy and emotional support in relationships. Joyful individuals are more attuned to the needs and feelings of their partners, friends, and family members, and they are better able to provide comfort and reassurance during difficult times.
   - Joy fosters a sense of compassion and understanding, allowing individuals to empathize with others' experiences and offer

genuine support and encouragement.

5. **Shared Goals and Values:**
   - Joyful relationships are often built on a foundation of shared goals, values, and interests. When individuals experience joy together, it strengthens their alignment and mutual understanding, leading to greater harmony and compatibility in relationships.
   - Shared experiences of joy create memories and traditions that deepen the bond between partners, friends, and family members, fostering a sense of connection and belonging.

6. **Conflict Resolution and Resilience:**

   - Joyful relationships are characterized by effective conflict resolution and resilience in the face of challenges. Joyful individuals approach conflicts with a sense of optimism and openness, seeking constructive solutions and maintaining a positive outlook on the relationship.

   - Shared experiences of joy serve as buffers against stress and adversity, helping couples and families navigate difficult times with grace and resilience.

7. **Fostering Gratitude and Appreciation:**

- Experiencing joy cultivates gratitude and appreciation in relationships. Joyful individuals express gratitude for their partners, friends, and family members, acknowledging their contributions and expressing love and affection.

- Gratitude and appreciation strengthen the bond between individuals, fostering a sense of mutual respect, admiration, and support in relationships.

8. **Promoting Playfulness and Fun:**

- Joyful relationships are characterized by playfulness, spontaneity, and fun. Couples and families who experience joy together engage in playful activities, shared hobbies, and adventures that bring laughter and excitement into their lives.

   - Playfulness fosters intimacy and connection between partners, friends, and family members, creating cherished memories and deepening the bond of love and affection.

9. **Creating a Positive Feedback Loop:**
   - Experiencing joy in relationships creates a positive feedback loop, where moments of joy reinforce and strengthen the connection between individuals. As relationships become more joyful

and fulfilling, they contribute to greater overall happiness and well-being for everyone involved.

   - The more joy individuals experience in their relationships, the more they invest in nurturing and sustaining those relationships, leading to greater satisfaction and fulfillment in the long term.

10. **Enhancing Relationship Satisfaction:**
   - Ultimately, the connection between joy and relationships enhances relationship satisfaction and fulfillment. Couples, families, and friends who experience joy together report higher levels of

happiness, intimacy, and overall well-being.

   - By prioritizing joy and cultivating positive emotions in relationships, individuals can create lasting bonds of love, support, and connection that enrich their lives and bring them greater happiness and fulfillment.

11. **Building Trust and Intimacy:**
   - Joyful relationships are characterized by trust and intimacy. When individuals experience joy together, it creates a sense of emotional safety and vulnerability, allowing them to open up and share their true selves with one another.

- Shared experiences of joy deepen the bond between partners, friends, and family members, fostering a sense of closeness and connection that strengthens the relationship over time.

12. **Promoting Forgiveness and Understanding:**
   - Experiencing joy in relationships promotes forgiveness and understanding. Joyful individuals are more likely to forgive mistakes and misunderstandings, recognizing that conflict is a natural part of any relationship.

- Shared experiences of joy help couples and families navigate conflicts with compassion and empathy, leading to greater understanding and acceptance of one another's imperfections.

13. **Supporting Personal Growth and Fulfillment:**
- Joyful relationships support personal growth and fulfillment. When individuals experience joy in their relationships, it encourages them to pursue their passions, dreams, and goals with the support and encouragement of their loved ones.
- Shared experiences of joy create a supportive environment

where individuals feel empowered to be their authentic selves and pursue their aspirations, leading to greater personal fulfillment and happiness.

14. **Creating a Sense of Belonging and Community:**
   - Experiencing joy in relationships creates a sense of belonging and community. Joyful individuals feel connected to their partners, friends, and family members, knowing that they have a supportive network of people who care about them and celebrate their successes.
   - Shared experiences of joy strengthen the sense of community

within relationships, fostering a supportive and nurturing environment where individuals feel valued, accepted, and loved.

15. **Bringing Balance and Harmony:**
   - Joyful relationships bring balance and harmony to individuals' lives. When individuals experience joy in their relationships, it creates a sense of equilibrium and fulfillment that extends to other areas of their lives.
   - Shared experiences of joy help individuals prioritize their relationships and invest time and energy in nurturing and sustaining

them, leading to greater overall life satisfaction and well-being.

Incorporating these additional aspects into our understanding of the connection between joy and enhancing relationships highlights the multifaceted nature of joyful relationships and their profound impact on individuals' lives. By prioritizing joy and cultivating positive emotions in relationships, individuals can create deep, meaningful connections with their loved ones and experience greater happiness, fulfillment, and well-being.

In summary, joy plays a central role in enhancing relationships by fostering connection, communication, empathy, shared goals, conflict resolution, gratitude, playfulness, and overall relationship satisfaction. By prioritizing joy and cultivating positive emotions in relationships, individuals can deepen their connections with loved ones and experience greater happiness and fulfillment in their interpersonal interactions.

"Chapter (4)"

Joy And Productivity

Increasing productivity often
involves a combination of

strategies and techniques. Here's a step-by-step guide to boosting productivity while fostering joy:

1. **Clarify Goals**: Clearly define your objectives and priorities. Knowing what you want to achieve helps direct your focus and efforts efficiently.

2. **Create a Positive Work Environment**: Surround yourself with elements that bring you joy, such as plants, photos, or inspiring quotes. A pleasant workspace can enhance your mood and motivation.

3. **Practice Mindfulness**: Incorporate mindfulness

techniques into your routine to stay present and focused. This can include meditation, deep breathing exercises, or simply taking short breaks to reset.

4. **Establish a Routine**: Develop a consistent daily routine that includes dedicated time for work, breaks, and self-care activities. Structure helps maintain productivity and reduces decision fatigue.

5. **Set Clear Boundaries**: Define boundaries between work and personal life to prevent burnout and maintain balance. Avoiding overwork can lead to greater

overall productivity and satisfaction.

6. **Prioritize Tasks**: Use techniques like the Eisenhower Matrix to categorize tasks based on urgency and importance. Focus on high-priority tasks first to maximize productivity.

7. **Break Tasks into Smaller Steps**: Break down larger projects into smaller, more manageable tasks. This approach makes it easier to tackle complex projects and reduces feelings of overwhelm.

8. **Utilize Time Management Techniques**: Experiment with techniques like the Pomodoro Technique, time blocking, or the 2-Minute Rule to enhance focus and productivity.

9. **Eliminate Distractions**: Identify and minimize sources of distraction in your environment, such as notifications, clutter, or noise. Consider using productivity tools or apps to help stay focused.

10. **Delegate and Collaborate**: Don't hesitate to delegate tasks or collaborate with others when appropriate. Sharing responsibilities we lighten your

workload and increase overall efficiency.

11. **Celebrate Progress**: Acknowledge and celebrate your achievements, no matter how small. Recognizing progress boosts morale and motivates continued productivity.

12. **Practice Gratitude**: Cultivate a mindset of gratitude by reflecting on positive aspects of your work and life. Gratitude enhances well-being and can increase overall satisfaction with your productivity efforts.

By integrating these steps into your daily routine, you can increase productivity while also nurturing a sense of joy and fulfillment in your work. Remember that productivity is not just about getting more done—it's also about finding joy and satisfaction in the process.

"Chapter (5)"

Joy And Resilience

Here's are detailed explanation of the connection between joy and resilience, in step by step:

1. **Understanding Joy**: Joy is a positive emotion characterized by feelings of happiness, contentment,

and satisfaction. It often arises from experiences that bring pleasure, fulfillment, or a sense of meaning.

2. **Impact on Well-being**: Experiencing joy has numerous benefits for mental and emotional well being. It can improve mood, reduce stress, boost immune function, and enhance overall quality of life.

3. **Building Resilience**: Resilience refers to the ability to adapt and bounce back from challenges, setbacks, and adversity. It involves developing coping skills, maintaining a positive

outlook, and fostering a sense of inner strength.

4. **Joy as a Coping Mechanism**: Joy can serve as a powerful coping mechanism during difficult times. so by staying with people that bring joy provides a temporary reprieve from stress and helps replenish emotional resources.

5. **Positive Emotions Broaden Thinking**: Research in positive psychology suggests that experiencing positive emotions, like joy, broadens individuals' cognitive and behavioral repertoires. This expanded thinking can facilitate

problem-solving and creativity, essential components of resilience.

6. **Enhancing Emotional Resources**: Regular experiences of joy contribute to the accumulation of emotional resources, such as optimism, gratitude, and self efficacy. These resources form the foundation of resilience, enabling individuals to navigate challenges with greater flexibility and effectiveness.

7. **Buffering Against Stress**: Joy acts as a buffer against the negative effects of stress. When individuals maintain a reservoir of positive emotions, they are better

equipped to withstand and recover from stressors, minimizing the risk of burnout or psychological distress.

8. **Promoting Social Connection**: Joyful experiences often occur in social contexts, such as spending time with loved ones or participating in group activities. Strong social connections serve as a key protective factor in resilience, providing emotional support, practical assistance, and a sense of belonging.

9. **Fueling Motivation and Purpose**: Joy can fuel intrinsic motivation and a sense of purpose,

which are essential components of resilience. When individuals derive joy from their work, relationships, or personal pursuits, they are more likely to persevere in the face of challenges and setbacks.

10. **Cultivating Gratitude and Appreciation**: Joy encourages individuals to cultivate gratitude and appreciation for the positive aspects of their lives. Gratitude practices have been linked to resilience by fostering a mindset of abundance, resourcefulness, and resilience.

11. **Embracing Moments of Joy**: In times of adversity, intentionally

seeking out and embracing moments of joy becomes especially important. Engaging in activities that evoke joy, such as hobbies, exercise, or spending time in nature, can provide a much needed source of resilience and renewal.

12. **Integration and Balance**: Ultimately, the connection between joy and resilience lies in their integration into daily life. By nurturing joy alongside resilience building practices, individuals can cultivate a robust emotional toolkit for navigating life's challenges with grace and strength.

By recognizing and nurturing the connection between joy and resilience, individuals can cultivate greater emotional well-being, adaptability, and capacity for thriving in the face of adversity.

"Chapter (6)"

Joy And Connection

This are step-by-step guide on how joy can improve communication:

1. **Understanding Joy**: Joy is a positive emotion characterized by feelings of happiness, satisfaction, and contentment. When individuals experience joy, it can influence various aspects of their behavior, including communication.

2. **Positive Emotional State**: Joy puts individuals in a positive emotional state, which can enhance communication by

fostering openness, warmth, and receptivity. When people are joyful, they are more likely to engage in interactions with enthusiasm and optimism.

3. **Facilitating Connection**: Joyfull communication can facilitate connection and rapport between individuals. Shared moments of joy create bonds and strengthen relationships, leading to more effective communication and collaboration.

4. **Nonverbal Cues**: Joy often manifests through nonverbal cues such as facial expressions, body language, and tone of voice. These

cues convey warmth, authenticity, and sincerity, making communication more engaging and impactfull.

5. **Enhanced Empathy**: Experiencing joy can enhance empathy and emotional intelligence, enabling individuals to better understand and respond to the emotions of others. This heightened empathy fosters deeper connections and more empathetic communication.

6. **Positive Energy**: Joy generates positive energy that is contagious in social interactions. When individuals communicate

joyfully, they radiate enthusiasm and vitality, uplifting the mood of those around them and creating a positive communication environment.

7. **Improved Listening**: Joyful communication promotes active listening and presence. When people are genuinely joyful, they are more attentive and responsive to others, leading to clearer understanding and more effective communication.

8. **Reduced Tension**: Joy has a calming effect on interpersonal dynamics, reducing tension and defensiveness in communication.

When individuals approach interactions with joy, they are less likely to engage in conflict or misinterpretation, fostering smoother communication flow.

9. **Promoting Creativity and Collaboration**: Joyful communication fosters a supportive and collaborative atmosphere conducive to creativity and innovation. When people feel joyful, they are more willing to share ideas, brainstorm solutions, and explore new possibilities together.

10. **Enhanced Problem-solving**: Joyful communication can enhance

problem solving by promoting a positive mindset and resilience in the face of challenges. When individuals approach communication with joy, they are more likely to focus on solutions rather than dwelling on problems, leading to more constructive outcomes.

11. **Building Trust**: Joyful communication builds trust and goodwill among communicators. When individuals express joy authentically, it signals transparency, honesty, and authenticity, strengthening trust and rapport in relationships.

12. **Creating Memorable Experiences**: Joyful communication leaves a lasting impression on participants, creating memorable experiences and deepening connections over time. When interactions are infused with joy, they become more meaningful and enriching, contributing to positive communication patterns in the long term.

By incorporating joy into communication practices, individuals can enhance connection, empathy, creativity, and trust in their interactions, fostering more fulfilling and effective relationships personally and professionally.

"Chapter (7)"

Promoting Longevity Through Joy

Increasing longevity through joy involves promoting a positive mindset, enhancing overall well-being, and adopting healthy lifestyle habits. Here's a detailed step-by-step guide:

1. **Understanding Joy and Longevity**: Joy is a positive emotion associated with happiness, contentment, and fulfillment. Research suggests that maintaining a joyful outlook on life can have a significant impact on longevity by reducing stress, promoting resilience, and fostering overall health.

2. **Positive Mindset**: Cultivate a positive mindset by focusing on gratitude, optimism, and appreciation for life's blessings.

Adopting a glass-half-full perspective can help reduce stress, boost immune function, and contribute to longevity.

3. **Stress Reduction**: Joyful experiences help counteract the negative effects of stress on the body. Engage in activities that bring you joy, such as spending time with loved ones, pursuing hobbies, or practicing mindfulness techniques like meditation or deep breathing exercises.

4. **Enhanced Immune Function**: Positive emotions, including joy, have been linked to enhanced

immune function. A strong immune system plays a crucial role in defending against illness and promoting longevity. Incorporate joyful activities into your daily routine to support overall immune health.

5. **Improved Cardiovascular Health**: Joyful experiences have been shown to benefit cardiovascular health by reducing blood pressure, improving heart rate variability, and promoting vascular health. Engage in joyful activities that get your heart pumping, such as dancing, walking

in nature, or participating in group exercise classes.

6. **Quality Relationships**: Cultivate meaningful relationships with family, friends, and community members. Strong social connections are associated with greater longevity and overall well-being. Spend time with loved ones, share joyful experiences, and prioritize nurturing your relationships.

7. **Sense of Purpose**: Find meaning and purpose in your life by pursuing activities that align with your values and passions. Having

a sense of purpose has been linked to increased longevity and better health outcomes. Identify what brings you joy and fulfillment, and incorporate these pursuits into your daily life.

8. **Healthy Lifestyle Habits**: Adopt healthy lifestyle habits that support longevity, such as maintaining a balanced diet, staying physically active, getting enough sleep, and avoiding harmful substances like tobacco and excessive alcohol. Joyful living encompasses taking care of your body and prioritizing your health.

9. **Resilience Building**: Joy promotes resilience, the ability to bounce back from adversity and navigate life's challenges with grace and strength. Cultivate resilience by embracing joy, practicing self-care, fostering positive relationships, and developing coping skills to manage stress effectively.

10. **Mind-Body Connection**: Recognize the interconnectedness of mind and body in promoting longevity. Joyful living involves nurturing both your mental and physical well-being through practices like mindfulness,

relaxation techniques, and engaging in activities that bring you joy and fulfillment.

11. **Continued Learning and Growth**: Stay curious, engaged, and open to new experiences throughout life. Lifelong learning and personal growth contribute to overall well-being and longevity. Explore new hobbies, pursue interests, and challenge yourself to continue growing and evolving.

12. **Gratitude and Appreciation**: Cultivate a mindset of gratitude and appreciation for the blessings in your life. Gratitude has been linked

to numerous health benefits, including increased longevity, improved sleep, and enhanced well-being. Take time each day to reflect on what you're grateful for and savor moments of joy and abundance.

By incorporating joy into your daily life and prioritizing habits that promote well-being, you can increase your chances of living a long, healthy, and fulfilling life. Joy serves as a powerful ally in promoting longevity by fostering resilience, reducing stress, and enhancing overall quality of life.

"Chapter (8)"

Joy And Quality Of Life

Certainly! The connection between joy and quality of life is multifaceted and deeply intertwined. Here's a step-by-step breakdown:

1. **Understanding Joy**: Joy is an intense feeling of happiness and satisfaction that arises from various sources such as fulfilling relationships, meaningful experiences, personal achievements, and sensory pleasures.

2. **Quality of Life Definition**: Quality of life encompasses various aspects of well-being, including physical health, mental and emotional well-being, social connections, financial stability,

environmental conditions, and overall life satisfaction.

3. **Impact of Joy on Mental Health**: Experiencing joy triggers the release of neurotransmitters such as dopamine, serotonin, and endorphins in the brain, which contribute to feelings of pleasure, contentment, and overall well-being. This positive impact on mental health is crucial for a high quality of life.

4. **Physical Health Benefits**: Joyful experiences and positive emotions have been linked to numerous physical health benefits, including reduced stress levels,

lower blood pressure, strengthened immune system, improved cardiovascular health, and increased longevity. These factors collectively contribute to an enhanced quality of life.

5. **Enhanced Coping Mechanisms**: Joy serves as a buffer against life's challenges and adversities. People who experience joy regularly tend to have better coping mechanisms, resilience, and adaptive strategies, which can significantly improve their quality of life, especially during difficult times.

6. **Positive Social Connections**: Joy is often shared with others

through laughter, celebrations, and bonding experiences. Strong social connections and meaningful relationships are fundamental components of quality of life, as they provide emotional support, a sense of belonging, and opportunities for personal growth and fulfillment.

7. **Sense of Purpose and Meaning**: Joy is closely tied to activities and pursuits that align with one's values, passions, and sense of purpose. Engaging in meaningful endeavors and experiences that bring joy can lead to a greater sense of fulfillment, satisfaction, and overall life

purpose, contributing to a higher quality of life.

8. **Long-Term Effects**: Cultivating joy and prioritizing activities that bring happiness and fulfillment can have long-term effects on overall quality of life. By fostering a positive outlook, nurturing relationships, pursuing passions, and practicing gratitude, individuals can create a foundation for sustained well-being and a fulfilling life.

9. **Alleviating Stress and Anxiety**: Joyful experiences have a natural stress-reducing effect on the body. When individuals

experience joy, they often experience a decrease in stress hormones like cortisol, leading to a sense of relaxation and ease. Over time, regularly experiencing joy can help reduce chronic stress and anxiety, leading to an overall improvement in quality of life.

10. **Promoting Creativity and Productivity**: Joy is often associated with a state of flow, where individuals are fully immersed and engaged in an activity they enjoy. This state of flow can foster creativity, innovation, and productivity. When individuals are engaged in activities that bring them joy, they are more

likely to perform at their best, leading to a sense of accomplishment and satisfaction, which in turn contributes to a higher quality of life.

11. **Improving Self-Confidence and Self-Esteem**: Joyful experiences can boost self-confidence and self-esteem by reinforcing a positive self-image. When individuals engage in activities that bring them joy and experience success or fulfillment in those activities, it can lead to a sense of competence and self-worth. This increased self-confidence and self-esteem can have far-reaching effects on

various aspects of life, including relationships, career, and personal development, ultimately enhancing overall quality of life.

12. **Promoting Physical Activity and Well-being**: Many joyful experiences involve physical activity, whether it's dancing, playing sports, or simply spending time outdoors in nature. Engaging in regular physical activity not only promotes physical health but also has numerous mental and emotional benefits, including improved mood, reduced stress, and enhanced cognitive function. By incorporating joyful physical activities into their routine,

individuals can improve their overall well-being and quality of life.

13. **Cultivating Gratitude and Appreciation**: Joy often arises from moments of gratitude and appreciation for the present moment and the blessings in one's life. Cultivating a practice of gratitude and mindfulness can amplify feelings of joy and contentment, leading to a greater sense of overall life satisfaction. By focusing on the positive aspects of life and expressing gratitude for them, individuals can shift their perspective and enhance their quality of life.

In essence, the connection between joy and quality of life is a reciprocal one, with joy contributing to various aspects of well-being and quality of life, and a high quality of life in turn creating the conditions for experiencing more joy. By prioritizing joy and actively seeking out experiences that bring happiness and fulfillment, individuals can significantly enhance their overall quality of life and well-being.

"Chapter (9)"

Joy And Motivation

Certainly! Increasing inspiration and motivation through joy involves cultivating a positive mindset, engaging in activities that bring joy, and harnessing the energy and enthusiasm generated by joyful experiences. Here's a step-by-step guide:

1. **Understanding Joy**: Joy is a positive emotion characterized by feelings of happiness, contentment, and fulfillment. It can arise from various sources, including

meaningful experiences, accomplishments, and connections with others.

2. **Identify Sources of Joy**: Reflect on activities, interests, and experiences that bring you joy. This could include spending time with loved ones, pursuing hobbies, engaging in creative outlets, or immersing yourself in nature.

3. **Set Meaningful Goals**: Identify goals and aspirations that resonate with your values and passions. Meaningful goals provide direction and purpose, fueling inspiration and motivation to take action.

4. **Visualize Success**: Visualize yourself achieving your goals and experiencing the joy and fulfillment that comes with success. Visualization techniques can enhance motivation by creating a vivid mental image of your desired outcome.

5. **Create a Joyful Environment**: Surround yourself with elements that evoke joy and inspiration, such as uplifting music, inspiring quotes, or artwork that resonates with you. A joyful environment can enhance creativity and motivation.

6. **Practice Gratitude**: Cultivate a mindset of gratitude by focusing on the positive aspects of your life and expressing appreciation for the blessings you have. Gratitude enhances well-being and fosters a sense of abundance, which can increase inspiration and motivation.

7. **Embrace Positive Self-Talk**: Monitor your internal dialogue and replace self-limiting beliefs with positive affirmations and encouragement. Positive self-talk boosts confidence, resilience, and motivation to pursue your goals.

8. **Seek Inspiration from Others**: Surround yourself with individuals

who inspire and motivate you. Engage with mentors, role models, or peers who embody qualities or achievements you aspire to. Their stories and insights can fuel your own inspiration and motivation.

9. **Practice Mindfulness**: Incorporate mindfulness practices into your daily routine to stay present and grounded. Mindfulness enhances awareness, clarity, and focus, providing a solid foundation for inspiration and motivation to flourish.

10. **Take Action Consistently**: Break down your goals into manageable steps and take

consistent action toward their realization. Momentum builds momentum, and each small achievement contributes to a sense of progress and momentum.

11. **Celebrate Successes**: Acknowledge and celebrate your achievements, no matter how small. Celebrating successes reinforces positive behaviors and motivates continued effort and progress.

12. **Reflect on Joyful Moments**: Reflect on moments of joy and fulfillment in your life. These memories serve as a source of inspiration and motivation,

reminding you of the joy that comes from pursuing your passions and living authentically.

By incorporating joy into your life and mindset, you can increase inspiration and motivation to pursue your goals and aspirations with enthusiasm and determination. Joy serves as a powerful catalyst for creativity, resilience, and personal growth, fueling a sense of purpose and fulfillment in your endeavors.

"Chapter (10)"

Joy And Emotional Regulations

Regulating emotions through joy involves harnessing positive feelings to manage and balance emotional responses effectively. Here's a step-by-step guide on how joy can help regulate emotions:

1. **Understanding Emotions**: Emotions are complex physiological and psychological responses to stimuli, influencing our thoughts, behaviors, and overall well-being. They range from positive emotions like joy and happiness to negative emotions like sadness and anger.

2. **Recognize Emotional Triggers**: Pay attention to situations, events, or thoughts that trigger emotional responses. Awareness of your emotional

triggers is the first step in regulating your emotions effectively.

3. **Cultivate Joy**: Engage in activities and practices that bring you joy and happiness. This could include spending time with loved ones, pursuing hobbies, practicing gratitude, or engaging in activities that evoke positive emotions.

4. **Practice Mindfulness**: Incorporate mindfulness techniques into your daily routine to stay present and aware of your emotions. Mindfulness helps you observe your emotions without judgment, allowing you to respond

to them in a more intentional and constructive manner.

5. **Savor Positive Experiences**: Take time to savor and fully experience moments of joy and happiness. Pay attention to the sensations, thoughts, and feelings associated with positive experiences, allowing them to uplift and regulate your emotions.

6. **Counter Negative Emotions**: Use joyful experiences to counteract and balance negative emotions. When you're feeling sad, anxious, or stressed, intentionally seek out activities or memories that

bring you joy to shift your emotional state.

7. **Express Gratitude**: Cultivate a mindset of gratitude by focusing on the positive aspects of your life. Expressing gratitude for the blessings you have can help regulate emotions by fostering a sense of abundance, appreciation, and contentment.

8. **Engage in Playfulness**: Embrace playfulness and humor as tools for regulating emotions. Playful activities and laughter can lighten your mood, reduce stress, and promote a sense of joy and well-being.

9. **Connect with Others**: Spend time with supportive and caring individuals who bring joy and positivity into your life. Social connections provide emotional support, companionship, and a sense of belonging, helping regulate emotions effectively.

10. **Set Boundaries**: Establish healthy boundaries in your relationships and daily life to protect your emotional well-being. Saying no to activities or interactions that drain your energy and saying yes to those that bring you joy and fulfillment can help

regulate your emotions more effectively.

11. **Practice Self-Compassion**: Treat yourself with kindness and compassion, especially during difficult times. Self-compassion involves acknowledging your emotions without judgment and responding to yourself with understanding and care.

12. **Seek Professional Help if Needed**: If you're struggling to regulate your emotions or experiencing significant emotional distress, don't hesitate to seek support from a therapist or counselor. Professional help can

provide you with strategies and tools to manage your emotions more effectively.

By incorporating joy into your life and utilizing positive emotions as tools for emotional regulation, you can cultivate greater resilience, well-being, and overall emotional balance. Joy serves as a powerful antidote to negative emotions, helping you navigate life's challenges with grace, positivity, and authenticity.

"Chapter (11)"

Joy And Social Connection

Certainly! The connection between joy and social connection is profound, as both concepts are intertwined and mutually reinforcing. Here's a step-by-step explanation of how joy enhances social connection:

1. **Understanding Joy**: Joy is a positive emotion characterized by feelings of happiness, contentment, and fulfillment. It arises from experiences that bring pleasure, satisfaction, or a sense of meaning.

2. **Social Nature of Joy**: Joy often occurs in social contexts, such as spending time with loved ones, celebrating achievements, or participating in group activities. Sharing joyful experiences with others amplifies the emotional impact and strengthens social bonds.

3. **Emotional Contagion**: Joy is contagious, spreading rapidly from one person to another through a phenomenon known as emotional contagion. When individuals experience joy, they naturally share their positive emotions with those around them, fostering a sense of connection and unity.

4. **Enhanced Communication**: Joyful individuals are more open, expressive, and engaging in their interactions with others. Positive emotions facilitate effective communication by promoting warmth, authenticity, and receptivity, which deepen social connections and rapport.

5. **Facilitating Empathy**: Experiencing joy enhances empathy and emotional intelligence, enabling individuals to better understand and respond to the emotions of others. Empathetic connections foster deeper relationships and mutual

understanding, strengthening social bonds.

6. **Building Trust and Intimacy**: Joyful interactions build trust and intimacy among participants, creating a safe and supportive environment for authentic expression and vulnerability. Trust is the foundation of meaningful relationships, and joy contributes to its cultivation.

7. **Shared Experiences**: Joyful experiences create shared memories and bonds that strengthen social connections over time. Whether it's celebrating milestones, overcoming

challenges, or simply enjoying each other's company, shared joy enhances the sense of belonging and solidarity within social groups.

8. **Promoting Cooperation and Collaboration**: Joy fosters a spirit of cooperation and collaboration among individuals, encouraging teamwork and mutual support. When people experience joy together, they are more inclined to work towards common goals and support each other's success.

9. **Alleviating Social Isolation**: Joyful interactions help alleviate feelings of social isolation and loneliness by providing

opportunities for meaningful connection and belonging. Regular social engagement and joyful experiences are essential for maintaining mental and emotional well-being.

10. **Strengthening Community Bonds**: Joyful communities are characterized by a sense of camaraderie, inclusivity, and supportiveness. Shared joy strengthens community bonds, fosters a sense of belonging, and promotes collective well-being.

11. **Promoting Positive Relationships**: Joyful individuals are more likely to attract positive

relationships and cultivate healthy social networks. Positive emotions serve as a magnet for like-minded individuals, leading to the formation of supportive friendships and social connections.

12. **Enhancing Overall Well-being**: The quality of social connections has a significant impact on overall well-being and life satisfaction. Joyful social interactions contribute to greater happiness, resilience, and fulfillment, enriching the fabric of life for individuals and communities alike.

By recognizing the connection between joy and social connection, individuals can prioritize activities and practices that foster positive emotions and meaningful relationships. Cultivating joy in social interactions strengthens bonds, promotes empathy, and enhances overall well-being, creating a ripple effect of positivity and connection in the world.

"Chapter (12)'

Joy Mindfulness And Presence

Certainly! The connection between joy and mindfulness/presence lies in their ability to cultivate awareness, deepen appreciation for the present moment, and enhance overall well-being. Here's a step-by-step explanation of this connection:

1. **Understanding Joy**: Joy is a positive emotion characterized by

feelings of happiness, contentment, and fulfillment. It arises from experiences that evoke pleasure, satisfaction, or a sense of meaning.

2. **Defining Mindfulness and Presence**: Mindfulness is the practice of paying deliberate attention to the present moment, with an attitude of openness, curiosity, and acceptance. Presence refers to being fully engaged and immersed in the current experience, free from distractions or preoccupation with the past or future.

3. **Awareness of Joyful Moments**: Mindfulness heightens

awareness of joyful moments as they unfold in the present moment. By tuning into our senses, thoughts, and emotions without judgment, we can fully appreciate the joy that arises from simple pleasures, meaningful connections, or moments of beauty.

4. **Deepening Gratitude and Appreciation**: Mindfulness cultivates gratitude and appreciation for the abundance of joy present in everyday life. By consciously observing and savoring moments of joy, we develop a deeper sense of gratitude for the blessings we often take for granted.

5. **Reducing Distraction and Ruminating Thoughts**: Mindfulness helps reduce distractions and ruminating thoughts that can hinder our ability to experience joy fully. By gently redirecting our attention back to the present moment, we can let go of worries about the past or future and immerse ourselves in the joy of the here and now.

6. **Embracing Impermanence**: Mindfulness encourages us to acknowledge the impermanent nature of joy and all human experiences. By accepting that joy, like all emotions, is transient and

ever-changing, we can fully embrace each moment of joy as it arises, without clinging or attachment.

7. **Cultivating Equanimity**: Mindfulness fosters equanimity, or a balanced and accepting attitude towards life's ups and downs. By developing equanimity, we can approach joy with a sense of calmness and non-attachment, appreciating it fully while recognizing that it is just one aspect of the human experience.

8. **Enhancing Emotional Resilience**: Mindfulness strengthens emotional resilience by

allowing us to observe and regulate our emotional responses more effectively. By practicing mindfulness, we can navigate difficult emotions with greater skill and cultivate a greater capacity to experience joy even in the midst of challenges.

9. **Fostering Presence in Relationships**: Presence enhances the quality of our relationships by allowing us to fully engage and connect with others. When we are fully present with loved ones, we can listen more deeply, communicate more authentically, and share moments of joy and connection more fully.

10. **Deepening Self-Compassion**: Mindfulness cultivates self-compassion by encouraging us to treat ourselves with kindness and acceptance, especially during moments of joy. By practicing self-compassion, we can fully embrace moments of joy without guilt or self-criticism, allowing ourselves to experience them more deeply.

11. **Nurturing Inner Peace**: Mindfulness and presence nurture inner peace by helping us find refuge in the present moment, free from worries or regrets. In the stillness of the present moment, we

can connect with a sense of inner joy and contentment that transcends external circumstances.

12. **Living with Intention and Purpose**: Mindfulness and presence empower us to live with intention and purpose, aligning our actions with our values and priorities. By bringing mindful awareness to our choices and behaviors, we can cultivate a life filled with joy, meaning, and fulfillment.

By integrating mindfulness and presence into our daily lives, we can deepen our connection with joy, cultivate a greater appreciation for the present moment, and enhance overall well-being. Mindfulness and presence serve as gateways to experiencing joy more fully and authentically, enriching our lives in profound and meaningful ways.

"Chapter (13)"

Joy And Creativity

Certainly! Enhancing creativity through joy involves fostering a positive mindset, cultivating an environment conducive to creative expression, and tapping into the inspiration and energy generated by joyful experiences. Here's a step by step guide:

1. What is Creativity? Creativity is the ability to generate new ideas, solutions, or expressions that are original, valuable, and meaningful. It encompasses a wide range of activities, including art, music, writing, problem solving, and innovation.

2. **Embracing Joyful Mindset**: Cultivate a positive and

open-minded mindset that embraces joy and curiosity. Approach creative endeavors with a sense of playfulness, enthusiasm, and wonder, allowing yourself to explore new possibilities without fear of judgment or failure.

3. **Tapping into Positive Emotions**: Joyful emotions, such as happiness, excitement, and inspiration, fuel creativity by enhancing mood, motivation, and cognitive flexibility. Engage in activities that bring you joy and uplift your spirits, whether it's spending time in nature, listening to music, or engaging in hobbies.

4. **Creating a Supportive Environment**: Surround yourself with elements that inspire creativity and evoke joy. This could include setting up a dedicated workspace filled with art supplies, inspirational quotes, or items that spark your imagination. A supportive environment encourages creative expression and experimentation.

5. **Mindful Exploration**: Practice mindfulness techniques to deepen your connection with the present moment and tap into your creative intuition. Mindfulness enhances awareness, clarity, and focus, allowing you to explore ideas and

insights with greater depth and insight.

6. **Embracing Playfulness**: Embrace a spirit of playfulness and experimentation in your creative process. Approach challenges with a sense of curiosity and wonder, allowing yourself to explore unconventional ideas and approaches without self-judgment or inhibition.

7. **Finding Inspiration in Joy**: Seek inspiration from joyful experiences and emotions. Pay attention to moments of joy and beauty in your daily life, drawing inspiration from nature, art,

relationships, or personal passions. Joyful experiences provide a rich source of inspiration for creative expression.

8. **Collaborative Creativity**: Engage in collaborative creative endeavors with others who share your joy and enthusiasm. Collaborative projects foster synergy, idea-sharing, and mutual support, leading to innovative solutions and dynamic creative outcomes.

9. **Embracing Failure as Learning**: Embrace failure as an inherent part of the creative process. View setbacks and

mistakes as opportunities for growth and learning, rather than obstacles to be avoided. Joyful creators approach challenges with resilience and optimism, using setbacks as stepping stones to success.

10. **Balancing Structure and Freedom**: Find a balance between structure and freedom in your creative process. While structure provides a framework for organizing ideas and executing plans, freedom allows for spontaneity, exploration, and improvisation. Joyful creators embrace both structure and

freedom, adapting their approach as needed to foster creativity.

11. **Celebrating Successes**: Celebrate your creative achievements, no matter how small. Acknowledge and honor your progress, milestones, and breakthroughs, reinforcing positive behaviors and fueling motivation to continue exploring and creating.

12. **Sharing Joy Through Creativity**: Share your creative gifts and talents with others, spreading joy and inspiration through your creations. Whether it's sharing artwork, music, writing, or innovative ideas, creative

expression has the power to uplift, inspire, and connect people in meaningful ways.

By incorporating joy into your creative process and mindset, you can enhance creativity, innovation, and self-expression. Joy serves as a catalyst for inspiration, motivation, and exploration, fueling a sense of wonder and possibility in your creative endeavors. Embrace joy as a guiding force in your creative journey, and watch as your creativity flourishes and evolves in exciting and unexpected ways.

"Chapter (14)"

Joy And Stress Reduction

Reducing stress through joy involves cultivating positive emotions, nurturing supportive relationships, and engaging in activities that promote relaxation and well-being. Here's a step-by-step guide:

1. **Understanding Stress**: Stress is a natural response to challenging or threatening situations, triggering physical, mental, and emotional reactions. Chronic stress can have

detrimental effects on health and well-being, making it important to manage effectively.

2. **Promoting Positive Emotions**: Joy is a positive emotion associated with feelings of happiness, contentment, and fulfillment. Cultivating joy and other positive emotions helps counteract the negative effects of stress by promoting relaxation, optimism, and resilience.

3. **Engaging in Joyful Activities**: Identify activities, hobbies, and experiences that bring you joy and fulfillment. Whether it's spending time with loved ones, pursuing

creative outlets, or connecting with nature, prioritize activities that uplift your spirits and promote a sense of well-being.

4. **Practicing Gratitude**: Cultivate a mindset of gratitude by focusing on the positive aspects of your life and expressing appreciation for the blessings you have. Gratitude reduces stress by shifting your focus from what's wrong to what's right, fostering a sense of abundance and contentment.

5. **Mindful Relaxation**: Practice mindfulness-based relaxation techniques to calm the mind and

body. Mindfulness meditation, deep breathing exercises, and progressive muscle relaxation promote relaxation, reduce tension, and alleviate stress symptoms.

6. **Nurturing Supportive Relationships**: Spend time with supportive and caring individuals who bring joy and positivity into your life. Strong social connections serve as a buffer against stress, providing emotional support, companionship, and a sense of belonging.

7. **Setting Boundaries**: Establish healthy boundaries in your relationships and daily life to

protect your well-being. Learn to say no to commitments or activities that drain your energy or contribute to stress, and prioritize self-care and relaxation instead.

8. **Finding Humor**: Incorporate humor and laughter into your daily life. Laughter triggers the release of endorphins, the body's natural feel-good chemicals, promoting relaxation and reducing stress levels.

9. **Spending Time in Nature**: Connect with nature to reduce stress and promote a sense of peace and tranquility. Spend time outdoors, go for walks in the park,

or engage in activities like gardening or birdwatching to rejuvenate your mind and body.

10. **Physical Activity**: Engage in regular physical activity to reduce stress and boost mood. Exercise releases endorphins, improves sleep quality, and provides a healthy outlet for pent-up energy and tension.

11. **Limiting Exposure to Stressors**: Identify and minimize exposure to sources of stress in your environment. This may involve setting boundaries with work, managing time effectively, and

avoiding situations or people that trigger stress reactions.

12. **Seeking Professional Help if Needed**: If stress becomes overwhelming or chronic, don't hesitate to seek support from a therapist or counselor. Professional help can provide you with strategies and coping skills to manage stress effectively and improve overall well-being.

By incorporating joy into your daily life and prioritizing activities and practices that promote relaxation and well-being, you can reduce stress levels and enhance your overall quality of life. Joy serves as a powerful antidote to stress, fostering resilience, optimism, and a greater sense of inner peace and contentment.

"Chapter (15)"

Joy And Fulfillment

Improving a sense of fulfillment through joy involves cultivating positive emotions, fostering meaningful connections, and pursuing activities aligned with personal values and passions. Here's a step-by-step guide:

1. **Understanding Fulfillment**: Fulfillment is a deep sense of satisfaction and contentment that arises from living a meaningful and purposeful life. It involves aligning one's actions, values, and goals with a sense of purpose and authenticity.

2. **Cultivating Positive Emotions**: Joy is a positive emotion that contributes to a sense of fulfillment by enhancing

happiness, contentment, and overall well-being. Cultivate joy by engaging in activities that bring you pleasure, satisfaction, and a sense of meaning.

3. **Mindful Presence**: Practice mindfulness to stay present and fully engaged in the moment. Mindfulness enhances awareness and appreciation of life's experiences, deepening your sense of fulfillment and connection to the present moment.

4. **Gratitude Practice**: Cultivate a mindset of gratitude by focusing on the positive aspects of your life and expressing appreciation for the

blessings you have. Gratitude promotes a sense of abundance, contentment, and fulfillment.

5. **Pursuing Passions**: Identify activities, hobbies, and interests that bring you joy and fulfillment. Pursue these passions with enthusiasm and dedication, allowing them to enrich your life and contribute to a sense of purpose and meaning.

6. **Setting Meaningful Goals**: Define personal goals and aspirations that align with your values and passions. Working towards meaningful goals provides a sense of direction and purpose,

enhancing your overall sense of fulfillment.

7. **Nurturing Relationships**: Cultivate meaningful connections with family, friends, and community members. Strong social connections provide support, companionship, and a sense of belonging, contributing to a deeper sense of fulfillment and well-being.

8. **Acts of Kindness**: Engage in acts of kindness and service to others. Helping others not only benefits those in need but also fosters a sense of connection, empathy, and fulfillment within yourself.

9. **Embracing Authenticity**: Embrace your true self and live authentically, aligning your actions with your values, beliefs, and passions. Authentic living promotes a sense of integrity, wholeness, and fulfillment.

10. **Finding Meaning in Challenges**: Embrace challenges and setbacks as opportunities for growth and learning. Overcoming obstacles and adversity can lead to a deeper sense of resilience, purpose, and fulfillment.

11. **Reflecting on Accomplishments**: Take time to

reflect on your accomplishments, no matter how small. Celebrate your successes and acknowledge the progress you've made towards your goals, reinforcing a sense of fulfillment and self-worth.

12. **Living with Intention**: Live with intention and purpose, making conscious choices that align with your values and aspirations. By living intentionally, you can create a life that is rich in meaning, fulfillment, and authenticity.

By incorporating joy into your daily life and prioritizing activities and relationships that bring you fulfillment, you can cultivate a deep sense of satisfaction, purpose, and meaning. Joy serves as a guiding force in your journey towards a more fulfilling and meaningful life, enriching your experiences and fostering a greater sense of well-being and contentment.

"Summary"

The Joy Prescription: Unlocking the Healing Power Within" by Abraham Hunter is a profound exploration into the transformative potential of joy as a catalyst for health, happiness, and fulfillment. Drawing upon scientific research, ancient wisdom, and personal insights, Hunter guides readers on a journey to discover the profound impact that joy can have on every aspect of our lives.

At its core, "The Joy Prescription" challenges conventional notions of wellness by presenting joy as the ultimate prescription for holistic health. Through a blend of compelling narratives, evidence-based research, and practical exercises, Hunter reveals how cultivating joy can enhance our physical, emotional, and spiritual well-being.

The book begins by examining the science behind joy, exploring how positive emotions stimulate the release of endorphins, boost the immune system, and promote overall longevity. Hunter delves into the interconnectedness of mind, body, and spirit, illustrating how joy acts as a powerful antidote to stress, anxiety, and disease.

Moving beyond the individual benefits of joy, Hunter explores its profound impact on relationships and community. He demonstrates how joyful individuals are more empathetic, compassionate, and resilient, fostering deeper connections and creating a ripple effect of positivity in their social circles.

"The Joy Prescription" also offers practical strategies for cultivating joy in daily life, providing readers with tools to embrace gratitude, mindfulness, and self-compassion. Through guided exercises and reflective prompts, Hunter empowers readers to awaken to the joy that lies within each moment and to reclaim their innate capacity for happiness and fulfillment.

Ultimately, "The Joy Prescription" is a call to action—a call to shift our focus from the pursuit of external achievements to the cultivation of inner joy. It invites readers to embark on a transformative journey of self-discovery, where they can tap into the boundless potential of joy and unlock the healing power that resides within their hearts.

By embracing joy as the ultimate prescription for health and happiness, readers will not only transform their own lives but also contribute to a world filled with compassion, connection, and vitality. "The Joy Prescription" is more than just a book; it is a roadmap to living a life of purpose, passion, and profound fulfillment.